QUICK CRITI

SUSAN B. STILLWELL, RN, MSN, CCRN

Cleveland Clinic Foundation,
Cleveland, Ohio

with 26 illustrations

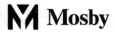 **Mosby**

St. Louis Baltimore Boston Chicago London Madrid
Philadelphia Sydney Toronto

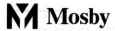
Mosby

Dedicated to Publishing Excellence

Publisher: Alison Miller
Editors: Terry Van Schaik; Timothy M. Griswold
Developmental Editor: Louann Morrow
Project Manager: Patricia Tannian
Production Editor: Barbara Jeanne Wilson
Designer: Gail Morey Hudson
Manufacturing Supervisor: John Babrick

SECOND EDITION
Copyright © 1994 by Mosby–Year Book, Inc.

Previous edition copyrighted 1990

Printed in the United States of America
Composition by Clarinda Company
Printing/binding by Plus Communications

Mosby–Year Book, Inc.
11830 Westline Industrial Drive, St. Louis, Missouri 63146

International Standard Book Number 0-8016-7693-2

95 96 97 / 9 8 7 6 5 4 3

CONTENTS

SECTION I ASSESSMENT GUIDES

I. VITAL SIGNS
A. *Temperature*

Conversion

To convert °F to °C: subtract 32 from °F, then multiply by 0.5555

To convert °C to °F: multiply °C by 1.8, then add 32

The Ws of Postoperative Fever

1. **WIND:** atelectasis—usually first 24-48 hours after surgery
2. **WEIN:** IV catheter—classic third day fever
3. **WATER:** urinary tract infection—usually occurs 5-8 days after Foley catheter inserted
4. **WOUND:** usually 6-10 days* after surgery
5. **WHERE:** positive intraabdominal abscesses—usually 7-14 days after surgery†
6. **WALKING:** thrombophlebitis in lower extremities—usually 7-14 days after surgery
7. **WONDER:** drug fever ("wonder drugs"—antibiotics?)

*β-hemolytic streptococci and clostridia can cause severe infections in 24-48 hours.

†From *pneumonic*—pus somewhere, pus nowhere (i.e., cannot find the pus), pus under the diaphragm.

B. *Pulse*

Classification of Pulse Strength

Value	Description
0	Absent
+1	Decreased, thready
+2	Normal
+3	Full, bounding

Variations in the arterial pulse (Figure 1)

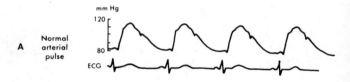

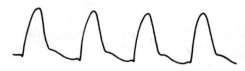

Fig. 1 Variations in arterial pulse.

C Small weak pulses, for example, cardiac shock

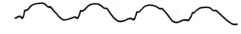

D Pulsus alternans, for example, congestive heart failure

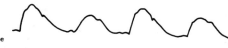

E Bigeminal pulse, for example, premature ventricular contractions

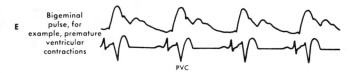

PVC

F Pulsus paradoxus, for example, pericardial tamponade

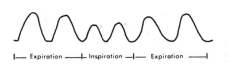

|— Expiration —|— Inspiration —|— Expiration —|

Fig. 1, cont'd.

3

C. *Respirations*

Respiratory Patterns

Pattern	
Eupnea	
Tachypnea	
Bradypnea	
Apnea	
Hyperpnea	
Cheyne-Stokes respiration	
Ataxic breathing	
Kussmaul's respiration	
Apneusis	
Obstructed breathing	

Rhythm is smooth and even with expiration longer than inspiration.

Rapid superficial breathing; regular or irregular rhythm; rate >20/min.

Slow respiratory rate; deeper than usual depth; regular rhythm; rate <12/min.

Cessation of breathing.

Increased depth of respiration with a normal to increased rate and regular rhythm; hyperventilation.

Periodic breathing associated with periods of apnea, alternating regularly with a series of respiratory cycles; the respiratory cycle gradually increases, then decreases in rate and depth.

Periods of apnea alternating irregularly with a series of shallow breaths of equal depth.

Deep regular sighing respirations with an increase in respiratory rate.

Long, gasping inspiratory phase followed by a short, inadequate expiratory phase.

Long, ineffective expiratory phase with shallow, increased respirations.

D. *Blood Pressure*

Auscultatory Gap (Figure 2)

Pulsus Paradoxus

Greater than 10 mm Hg fall in systolic blood pressure (SBP) during inspiration. Associated with acute cardiac tamponade, constrictive pericarditis, severe obstructive lung disease.

- Inflate BP cuff above known systolic pressure
- Slowly deflate cuff (patient should be breathing normally)
- Note when first sounds are heard during expiration
- Continue deflating cuff
- Note when sounds begin again and are heard continuously during respiratory cycle
- Continue deflating cuff until sounds disappear

The difference between the first sound and the continuous sound is the pulsus paradoxus.

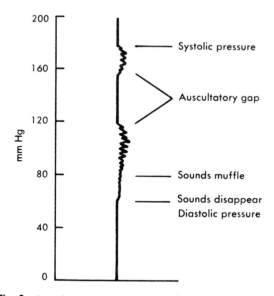

Fig. 2 Auscultatory gap. Systolic sounds are first heard at 180 mm Hg. They disappear at 160 mm Hg and reappear at 120 mm Hg; silent interval is auscultatory gap. Korotkoff sounds muffle at 80 mm Hg and disappear at 60 mm Hg. Blood pressure is recorded as 180/80/60 with auscultatory gap. If cuff was inflated to 150 mm Hg, reading may be interpreted as normotensive, when in fact patient is hypertensive.

II. NEUROLOGIC
A. *Level of Consciousness*

Glasgow Coma Scale

Eyes open	
spontaneously	4
to command	3
to pain	2
no response	1
Motor response	
obeys command	6
localizes pain	5
withdraws	4
flexion (abnormal)	3
extension (abnormal)	2
no response	1
Verbal response	
oriented	5
confused	4
inappropriate words	3
incomprehensible sounds	2
no response	1

Scores <7 are defined as coma.

B. *Terminology*

Localizes pain: reaches toward and removes stimulus

Withdrawal: pulls extremity or body away from stimulus

Flexion (decorticate): arms (one or both) flexed over chest; legs may be extended (Figure 3)

Extension (decerebrate): arms (one or both) extended; legs may be extended (Figure 3)

Flaccid: no response

C. *Posturing* (Figure 3)

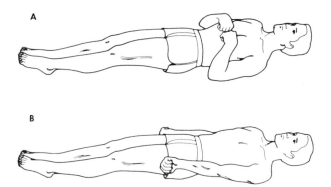

Fig. 3 A, Flexion or decorticate rigidity. **B,** Extension or decerebrate rigidity.

D. *Pupils*

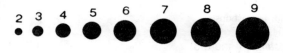

Fig. 4 Pupil Gauge (mm).

E. *Motor Function*

Scale for Muscle Movement of Extremities

Score	Movement
0	No contraction
1	Slight flicker/trace of contraction
2	Active (gravity eliminated)
3	Active; against gravity but not against resistance
4	Active; against gravity and resistance but not full strength
5	Full strength against examiner's resistance

F. *Reflexes*

Scale for Deep Tendon Reflexes

Score	Description
0	Absent
1+	Diminished
2+	Normal
3+	Increased, more brisk than average
4+	Hyperactive, clonus

Babinski—dorsiflexion of the big toe and fanning of the toes when sole of foot is stroked. Positive reflex = upper motor neuron dysfunction.

Oculocephalic (doll's eye maneuver)—reflex tested in the unconscious patient to determine intact brainstem pathways. If reflex is absent, patient may not be able to protect the airway via gag and cough reflexes.

Intact reflex: eyes remain in the initial position, then turn slowly to the direction in which the head was rotated.

Absent reflex: eyes move with the head as though fixed in place.

Oculovestibular (ice water calorics)

Normal (in conscious person): nystagmus, with slow movement toward the irrigated ear and rapid movement away.

Supratentorial or metabolic lesion: eyes move slowly toward irrigated ear and remain there for 2-3 minutes. The fast return to midline is absent.

Brainstem lesion: downward deviation and rotary jerking of one eye.

Severe brainstem damage: absent caloric response.

G. *Evaluating a Seizure*

Onset: sudden, aura

Duration: length of seizure activity

Activity: how it begins, progresses; what body parts are involved and type of movement; any tongue or eye deviation

LOC: during seizure, after seizure, duration of unconsciousness after seizure

Pupils: size, reaction, deviation

Respirations: apnea, cyanosis

Elimination: incontinent of urine/feces

III. PULMONARY

A. *Auscultation* (Figure 5)

B. *Respiratory Terms*

Fine crackles: similar to rubbing strands of hair together next to the ear

Coarse crackles: bubbling quality similar to carbonated soda

Rhonchi: snoring quality, continuous, similar to rubbing 2 inflated balloons together

Wheeze: musical quality, continuous

Pleural friction rub: leathery, creaking sound heard during inspiration and expiration

Bronchophony: "99" or "66" is heard distinctly with consolidation

Egophony: "E" sounds like "A" with consolidation or pleural effusion

Whispered pectoriloquy: "1,2,3" (when whispered by patient) is clearly auscultated with consolidation

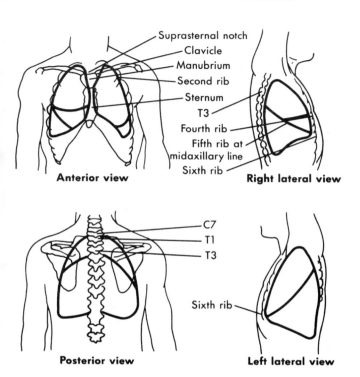

Anterior view

Suprasternal notch
Clavicle
Manubrium
Second rib
Sternum
T3
Fourth rib
Fifth rib at
midaxillary line
Sixth rib

Right lateral view

Posterior view

C7
T1
T3

Sixth rib

Left lateral view

Fig. 5 Location of lobes of lung using anatomical landmarks.

C. Quick Guide to Evaluate a Chest Film

Structure	Normal
Trachea	Midline position
Clavicles	Equidistant from sternum
Hilum	White densities where bronchi join lungs; left hilum is 2-3 cm higher than right hilum
Heart	Cardiothoracic ratio <50%
Lungs	Radiolucent
Diaphragm	Right side is 1-2 cm higher than left; should be rounded structures
Costophrenic angles	Clear and sharp

Abnormal Radiographic Findings

Finding	Possible Diagnosis
Nondistinct or widened aortic knob	Aortic dissection
Silhouette sign (loss of border visibility)	Infiltrates or consolidation RML or lingula
Blackened area	Pneumothorax
Patchy infiltrates or streaky densities	Pneumonia, atelectasis
Fluffy infiltrates (Kerley B lines)	Pulmonary edema
Loss of costophrenic angle sharpness	Pleural effusion

D. *Oxygenation*

Blood Gases: Normal Values

Arterial		Venous
7.35-7.45	pH	7.31-7.41
80-100 mm Hg	pO_2*	30-40 mm Hg
35-45 mm Hg	pCO_2	41-51 mm Hg
21-25 mEq/L	HCO_3	22-29 mEq/L
95%-99%	O_2 sat	60%-85%
−2 to +2	BE	0 to +4

*In a patient >60 years old, PaO_2 is equal to 80 mm Hg minus 1 mm Hg for every year over 60. Expected PaO_2 =FiO_2 × 5

Interpreting ABGs

1. Check pH   ↑ = alkalosis; ↓ = acidosis
2. Check pCO_2 ↑ = CO_2 retention (hypoventilation); respiratory acidosis or compensating for metabolic alkalosis

                  ↓ = CO_2 blown off (hyperventilation); respiratory alkalosis or compensating for metabolic acidosis

3. Check HCO_3 ↑ = nonvolatile acid is lost; HCO_3 gained (metabolic alkalosis or compensating for respiratory acidosis)

                  ↓ = nonvolatile acid is added; HCO_3 is lost (metabolic acidosis or compensating for respiratory alkalosis)

4. Determine imbalance
5. Determine if compensation exists

Determining the Imbalance in ABGs

If

$pH \uparrow$ and $pCO_2 \downarrow$
    or
$pH \downarrow$ and $pCO_2 \uparrow$
} Then respiratory disorder

If

$pH \uparrow$ and $HCO_3 \uparrow$
    or
$pH \downarrow$ and $HCO_3 \downarrow$
} Then metabolic disorder

If

$pCO_2 \uparrow$ and $HCO_3 \uparrow$
    or
$pCO_2 \downarrow$ and $HCO_3 \downarrow$
} Then compensation is occurring

If

$pCO_2 \uparrow$ and $HCO_3 \downarrow$
    or
$pCO_2 \downarrow$ and $HCO_3 \uparrow$
} Then mixed imbalance

SvO_2 Monitoring

Reflects O_2 supply/demand status. NOTE: maintain patency of the catheter. Placement of catheter outside the PA can result in inaccurate measurements.

Normal: 60%-80%

Abnormal low:

Cause: patient using venous reserve, inability to increase supply to match demand

Examples: $\downarrow$ CO, $\downarrow$ Hgb, $\downarrow$ SaO_2, and $\uparrow$ in tissue demand (suctioning, toileting, weighing patient)

Abnormal high:

Cause: impaired cellular use of O_2, oxyhemoglobin dissociation curve shift to the left

Examples: sepsis, cyanide toxicity, hypothermia, alkalosis

Significant readings:

Changes >10%

or S_vO_2 < 60% warrants an examination of the patient

e.g. cardiac output, ABGs, hemoglobin level

E. *Intubation/Extubation Guidelines*

Intubation

Tube size:

Orotracheal	*Nasotracheal*
males: 8-8.5 mm i.d.	<7.5 mm i.d.
females: 7-8 mm i.d.	

Cuff pressure:

>20 mm Hg increases risk for tracheal damage

<15 mm Hg increases risk of aspiration around cuff

Ventilation:

Auscultate the lateral aspect of the chest midaxillary line for presence of breath sounds.

Inspect chest for equal expansion.

Auscultate over the epigastric area. Gurgling sounds indicate esophageal intubation—remove tube and reintubate.

Minimal occlusive technique:

Place stethoscope at larynx

Slowly remove air (in 0.2 ml amounts) from cuff until air leak is heard

Slowly reinsert air (in 0.2 ml amounts) until the inspiratory leak stops

Stabilize tube:

Mark depth of tube and check periodically for displacement

Avoid excessive negative pressure when suctioning (-80 to -120 mm Hg)

Support ventilator tubing when moving/suctioning patient

Avoid unnecessary tube manipulation

Avoid unnecessary suctioning

Sedate patient prn to decrease risk of self-extubation

Extubation

Elevate HOB

Preoxygenate (100%)

Suction endotracheal tube, above tube cuff, from patient's mouth

Instruct patient to take in a deep breath; deflate cuff and remove tube on peak inspiration

Administer prescribed oxygen

Assess signs and symptoms indicative of respiratory distress and increased effort

Signs and Symptoms Indicative of Respiratory Distress and Increased Effort

If pulse ↑ or ↓ by 20 bpm or <60

If BP ↑ or ↓ by 20 mm Hg

If RR >30 or <8

If PAWP >20 mm Hg

Other findings: dyspnea, panic, fatigue, cyanosis, dysrhythmias, nasal flaring, intercostal retractions, altered breathing pattern, paradoxical motion of rib cage and abdomen

F. *Mechanical Ventilation*

Parameter and normal value	Criteria for weaning
Vital capacity (65-75 ml/kg)	>10-15
Tidal volume (5-7 ml/kg)	>5
Respiratory rate (12-20 breaths/min)	12-20
Minute ventilation (5-6 L/min)	<10
Negative inspiratory force (-75 to -100 cm H_2O)	>-25
$PaCO_2$ (35-45 mm Hg)	<45 (except COPD patients)
PaO_2 (80-100 mm Hg)	>70 on FiO_2 40%
FEV_1 (50-60 ml/kg)	>16
V_D/V_T (<0.3)	<0.6

G. *Troubleshooting the Ventilator*

Alarm	Assessment
High pressure or peak pressure	CHECK: Ventilator tubing and eliminate kinks Ventilator tubing for water accumulation and empty For secretions and suction prn ET tube placement If patient biting ET tube or bucking ventilator
Volume or pressure	CHECK: If patient disconnected from ventilator For decrease in patient's initiated breaths For leak around ET cuff ET tube placement For loose connections

H. *Chest Tube Drainage*

Collection Chamber/Drainage

If >100 ml/h ×2, notify MD

If decreased, check for kinks, clots (milking tube is controversial)

Water Seal Chamber

Add/remove fluid prn. Fluid level is usually 2-3 cm.

Check fluctuations (tidaling); if excessive, may indicate distress; if decreased, may indicate an obstruction or reexpansion of lung (fluid moves upward on inspiration and downward on expiration; if on a positive pressure ventilator, the opposite occurs).

Check for continuous bubbles (air leak in system or massive air leak from patient). If unexpected bubbling occurs, clamp tube near patient. If bubbling stops, the leak is at the insertion site or inside the patient; notify MD. If bubbling does not stop, the leak is in the system. Localize the leak by clamping the tube along the system. Replace tube, retape connections or replace the device.

Suction Control Chamber (Usually 15-25 cm Water)

Check fluid level—this level regulates the amount of suction.

Check bubbling—avoid vigorous bubbling; maintain constant but gentle bubbling.

IV. CARDIOVASCULAR

A. *Estimating Central Venous Pressure* (Figure 6)

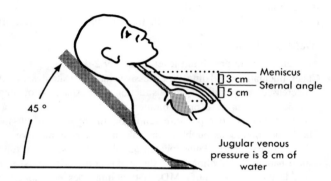

Fig. 6 Estimation of central venous pressure. Identify highest level of pulsations in internal jugular vein (meniscus). Determine vertical distance between sternal angle and meniscus. Add that distance to constant 5 cm (sternal angle is 5 cm above mid-RA level).

B. *Scale for Pitting Edema*

Value	Description
+1	5 mm depth
+2	8-10 mm depth
+3	>10 mm depth, lasting up to 30 sec
+4	>20 mm depth, lasting longer than 30 sec

C. *Auscultation* (Figure 7)

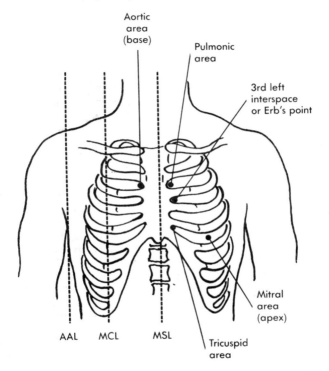

Fig. 7 Cardiac auscultatory sites. S_1 is heard loudest at mitral and tricuspid areas. S_2 is heard loudest at aortic and pulmonic areas. S_3 and S_4 are heard best at mitral area.

D. *Heart Sounds* (Figure 8)

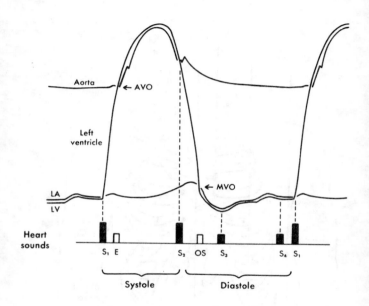

Fig. 8 Normal and abnormal heart sounds during one complete cardiac cycle as correlated with left-sided heart pressure waves. Right-sided heart pressures have been omitted for simplification. At onset of ventricular systole, left ventricular *(LV)* pressure exceeds left atrial *(LA)* pressure to close mitral valve, producing S_1 (in association with tricuspid valve closure.) When LV pressure exceeds aortic pressure, aortic valve opens *(AVO)*. With valvular disease and hypertension, aortic valve opening may be audible and heard as early ejection click *(E)*. When aortic pressure exceeds LV pressure, aortic valve closes to produce S_2 in association with pulmonic valve closure. When LV pressure drops below LA pressure, mitral valve opens *(MVO)*. With thickening of mitral valve as result of rheumatic heart disease, opening snap *(OS)* is produced in early diastole. During rapid ventricular filling an S_3, or ventricular gallop, is produced in patients with myocardial failure. Late in diastole, S_4, or atrial gallop, is produced in association with atrial contraction, owing to increased resistance to ventricular filling.

E. Scale for Grading Murmurs

Grade	Description
I	Soft, barely audible
II	Audible, quiet
III	Moderately loud, no thrill
IV	Loud, no thrill
V	Very loud, associated with a thrill
VI	Very loud, associated with a thrill; heard with a stethoscope off the chest

V. GI/METABOLIC (Figure 9)

A. *Bowel Sounds*

Normal: 3-35 sounds/minute

Increased: early intestinal obstruction

Decreased: peritonitis, paralytic ileus, electrolyte imbalance

B. *Guide to NG Tube Placement*

1. Measure NEX: from bridge of nose to ear lobe to xiphoid process
2. Check placement by:
   - Aspirating gastric contents
   - Auscultating for rush of air over gastric area when injecting air
   - Placing end of tube in water and checking for bubbling (indicates tube is in bronchus)
3. Confirm placement with X-ray examination

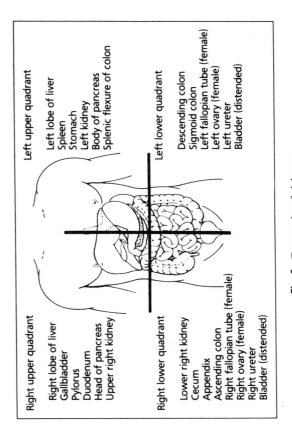

Right upper quadrant

Right lobe of liver
Gallbladder
Pylorus
Duodenum
Head of pancreas
Upper right kidney

Left upper quadrant

Left lobe of liver
Spleen
Stomach
Left kidney
Body of pancreas
Splenic flexure of colon

Right lower quadrant

Lower right kidney
Cecum
Appendix
Ascending colon
Right fallopian tube (female)
Right ovary (female)
Right ureter
Bladder (distended)

Left lower quadrant

Descending colon
Sigmoid colon
Left fallopian tube (female)
Left ovary (female)
Left ureter
Bladder (distended)

Fig. 9 Topography of abdomen.

VI. FLUID AND ELECTROLYTES

A. *Fluid Volume Assessment*

Parameter	Hypovolemia	Hypervolemia
Weight	Acute loss	Acute gain
Pulse	Tachycardia	Bounding
BP	Postural hypotension, decreased pulse pressure	Hypertension
Mucous membranes	Dry	Moist
Turgor	Decreased skin elasticity, furrowed tongue	Pitting edema
Peripheral veins	Jugular vein flat when supine; slow filling hand veins	Jugular vein distended
Hemodynamics	CVP <2 cm H_2O ↓ PAWP	CVP >12 cm H_2O ↑ PAWP
Other	Thirst, u/o <30 ml/hr	Cough, dyspnea, crackles, S_3, pulmonary edema
Laboratory	↑ hemoglobin ↑ hematocrit ↑ serum osmolality ↑ specific gravity ↑ BUN:creatinine ratio	↓ hemoglobin ↓ hematocrit ↓ serum osmolality ↓ specific gravity

B. *Electrolyte Imbalances*

Imbalance	Signs and symptoms
↓ Na	Hypotension, tachycardia, headache, dizziness, weakness, lethargy, restlessness, confusion, delirium, muscle tremors, convulsions, ataxia, aphasia, anorexia, nausea/vomiting, abdominal cramps, paralytic ileus
↑ Na	Lethargy, disorientation, muscle rigidity, tremors, spasms, hyperactive reflexes, irritability, coma, cerebral hemorrhage, hypotension, dry skin, dry mucous membranes, fever
↓ K	Dysrhythmias, depressed S-T segment, flattened or inverted T wave, increased amplitude of P wave, prolonged P-R interval, widened QRS complex; postural hypotension; confusion, lethargy, apathy, drowsiness, irritability, delirium; muscle weakness, paralysis; abdominal distention, constipation, paralytic ileus, frequent voiding, thirst
↑ K	Muscle weakness; cardiotoxicity; ECG changes include high, peaked T wave, prolonged P-R interval, absent P waves, widened QRS complex
↓ Mg	Confusion, restlessness, irritability, vertigo, seizures; muscle tremors, carpopedal spasm, nystagmus, spasticity; tachycardia, hypotension, PACs, PVCs
↑ Mg	Muscle weakness, paralysis; cardiac dysrhythmias, hypotension; respiratory insufficiency; drowsiness, lethargy, coma

SECTION II MONITORING GUIDELINES

I. ARTERIAL LINE
A. *Allen Test:*

Perform Allen test before placement of arterial line.

B. *Transducer Placement:*

Place at phlebostatic axis (Figure 10) or tip of intraarterial catheter. Use consistency in transducer placement to obtain readings.

C. *Waveform:*

Check waveform appearance (Figure 11).

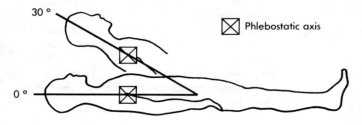

30°   ☒ Phlebostatic axis

0°

Fig. 10 Phlebostatic axis.

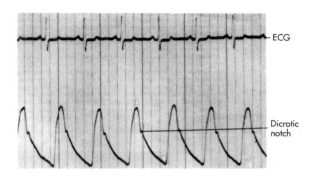

Fig. 11   Arterial waveform with corresponding ECG.

II. PULMONARY ARTERY CATHETER

Proximal port is for measuring CVP or may be used for infusions; distal port is used to measure pulmonary artery pressures and is not recommended for infusions.

A. *Normal Values:*

PAS	15-30 mm Hg
PAD	5-15 mm Hg
PAM	10-20 mm Hg
PAWP	4-12 mm Hg
RA (CVP)	0-8 mm Hg
RV	$\frac{15\text{-}28}{0\text{-}8}$ mm Hg

B. *Transducer Placement:*
Phlebostatic axis (Figure 10); HOB <30°

C. *Waveform* (Figure 12)

D. *Cautions:*
- Read pressure at end expiration
- Avoid inflating balloon with fluid
- Allow balloon to deflate passively
- Avoid overinflation of balloon
- Avoid balloon inflation greater than 15 sec
- Avoid flushing line in PAWP position

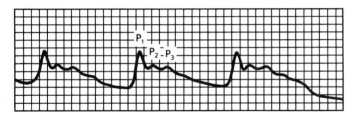

Fig. 13 ICP waveform.

C. *Transducer Placement*

The foramen of Monro is the reference point (Figure 14). The outer canthus of the eye or top of ear or external auditory meatus can also be used.

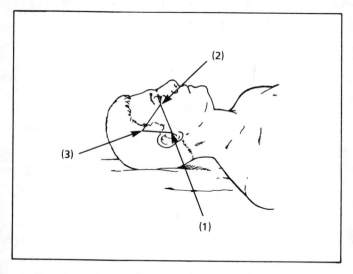

Fig. 14 Location of foramen of Monro for transducer placement. Map an imaginary equilateral triangle from (1) the external auditory meatus, to (2) the outer canthus of the eye, to (3) behind the hairline. Point 3 is the location of the foramen of Monro.

V. CHECKLIST FOR ICP MONITORING

Problem	Action
No waveform	Check power to monitor and to trace
	Check gain setting
	Check all connections
	Check for air bubbles in system
	NOTE: Only flush intraventricular catheter or screw under direction of MD
High pressure reading	Check transducer level placement
	Check calibration and rezero
	Evaluate patient:
	Check airway
	Check ventilator settings
	Check ABGs for hypoxemia, hypercarbia
	Check HOB (15-30 degrees)
	Check position of head (do not rotate head)
	Check extremities (limit flexion in lower extremities and hips)
	Check excessive muscle activity (administer muscle relaxants, paralyzing agents as ordered)
	Check abdominal distention
	Check noxious stimuli and remove
	Check temperature
	Check PAP, CO, SvO_2, BP
	Check electrolytes

Problem	Action
Low pressure reading	Check transducer level placement (Figure 14) Check for otorrhea and rhinorrhea Check for dislodged catheter—notify MD Check if 15-20 mm Hg positive pressure exists (with use of external ventriculostomy)

VI. IABP
A. *Waveform Analysis* (Figure 15)
   1. Identify the beginning of systole—balloon deflation occurs at end diastole.
   2. Identify the beginning of diastole—balloon inflation occurs at the dicrotic notch.
   3. Inflation and deflation are triggered by the R wave of the ECG tracing.

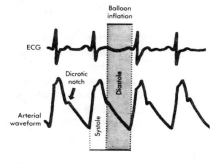

Fig. 15 IABP period of balloon inflation.

B. *Proper Inflation* (Figure 16)

1. Identify the dicrotic notch of the arterial tracing. The U shape of the patient's unassisted beat *A* should change to a V shape in the assisted beat *B* (Figure 16).

C. *Proper Deflation* (Figure 16)

1. Compare end-diastolic pressures 1 and 2. 1 should be lower than 2. At least 5-15 mm Hg difference is desirable.
2. Compare the systolic peak pressures 3 and 4. The balloon assisted systole 3 should be < the patient's systolic pressure 4.

D. *IABP Weaning Criteria*

CI $\geq$ 2 L/min/m^2
PAWP <18-20 mm Hg
SBP $\geq$100 mm Hg
U/O $\geq$30 ml/hr
Absence of crackles, S$_3$

Improved mentation
Absence of life-threatening
   dysrhythmias
Absence of ischemia on ECG
HR <110 bpm

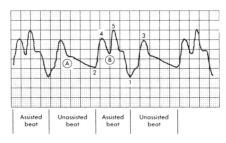

Fig. 16 IABP waveform. *1*, Balloon-assisted end diastolic pressure; *2*, patient's end diastolic pressure; *3*, "assisted" systole (occurs after balloon assisted beat); *4*, patient's systolic pressure; *5*, peak diastolic pressure (augmented diastolic pressure).

ELECTROCARDIOGRAPHY

I. MONITOR LEADS

	MCL$_1$ (V$_1$)	MCL$_6$ (V$_6$)	II*
Positive electrode	V$_1$ position 4th ICS, RSB	V$_6$ position 5th ICS, MAL	Below rib cage, left lower torso
Negative electrode	Below L clavicle	Below L clavicle	Below R clavicle
Ground	Below R clavicle	Below R clavicle	Below L clavicle

*Lead II is inadequate for distinguishing SVT with BBB or aberration from VT.

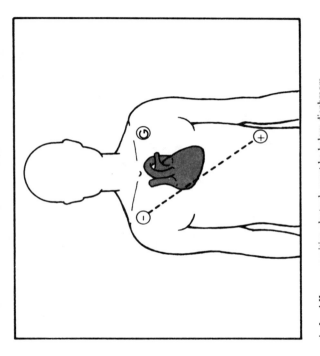

A, Lead II. NOTE: positive electrode must be below diaphragm.

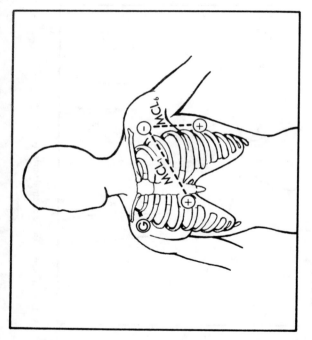

B, Lead MCL1 and MCL6.

Ideal Monitoring Leads

Problem to assess	Lead
Wide QRS rhythms	MCL_1; MCL_6 if MCL_1 not practical
	$MCL_1 - MCL_6$ combination if dual chamber monitor available
	V_1, I, aVF if three ECG channels available
New BBB	V_1 or MCL_1
	MCL_6 if MCL_1 not practical
Ischemia	Check ECG leads for ST changes before thrombolytic therapy or during PTCA
	Use MCL_1 if any ST changes occur in V_1; V_2 or V_3 for monitoring LAD coronary artery;
	III for monitoring circumflex artery; III or aVF for monitoring right coronary artery

II. MEASURING HEART RATE AND RHYTHM
A. *Heart Rate*
1. Count the number of R waves in a 6-sec strip and multiply by 10.
2. Count the number of large boxes between 2 R waves and divide into 300 (Figure 17).
3. Count the number of small boxes between 2 R waves and divide into 1500 (Figure 17).

NOTE: If heart rhythm is irregular, use method 1.

B. *Rhythm*
1. Measure R-R interval; if the difference between the shortest R-R and longest R-R intervals is >0.12, the rhythm is irregular.

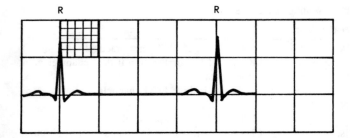

Fig. 17 Rate calculations using methods 2 and 3. Method 2: count number of large boxes between two R waves and divide into 300, i.e., 300 ÷ 4 large boxes = 75 bpm. Method 3: count number of small boxes between two R waves and divide into 1500, i.e., 1500 ÷ 20 small boxes = 75 bpm.

C. Criteria for a Normal Electrocardiogram

Component	Criteria
Rhythm	Atrial and ventricular are same; R-R and P-P intervals vary less than 0.16 sec
Rate	Atrial and ventricular rates are equal; 60-100 cycles/min
P wave	Present; only one P for each QRS
Direction	Upright in I, II, aVF, and V_4 to V_6; inverted in aVR; biphasic, flat or inverted in III, V_1, and V_2
	Upright and notched in I, II, V_4 to V_6 suggests left atrial abnormality
Shape	Rounded, symmetrical, without notches, peaks
Amplitude	<3.0 mm

Component	Criteria
Width	1.5 to 2.5 mm (0.06-0.10 sec)
	Tall and peaked in II, III, aV_F suggests lung disease
Axis	0 to +90 degrees
PR interval	0.12 to 0.20 sec
	>0.20 = AVB
QRS interval	0.06 to 0.10 sec
	>0.12 = BBB
	V_1, V_2 are best to measure QRS
QT interval	<Half the preceding R-R interval in normal rates
	$$Q\text{-}Tc = \frac{Q\text{-}t \text{ (measured)}}{\sqrt{R\text{-}R \text{ interval(s)}}}$$
	Normal = 0.30 − 0.40 sec
	Prolonged QT interval is associated with torsade de pointes
QRS complex	Follows each P
Configuration	Upper- and lower-case letters indicate the relative sizes of the QRS components.

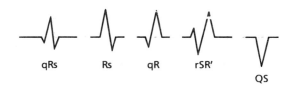

qRs   Rs   qR   rSR′   QS

Continued.

Component	Criteria
ST segment	Isoelectric, but may be elevated <1 mm in limb leads and <2 mm in some precordial leads
	Not depressed more than 0.05 mm
	Curves gently into proximal limb of T wave
	Elevation associated with vasospasm or acute injury; depression suggests ischemia
T-wave	
Direction	Upright in I, II, and V_3 to V_6; inverted in aVR; and varies in III, aVL, aVF, V_1 and V_6
Shape	Slightly rounded and asymmetrical
Height	<5 mm in limb leads; <10 mm in precordial leads
	Tall T wave is associated with hyperkalemia, ischemia
Axis	Left and inferior
Q wave	Width: <0.039 sec
	Significant if 0.04 sec
	Depth: 1-2 mm in I, aVL, aVF, V_5 and V_6; deep QS or Qr in aVR and possibly in III, V_1, and V_2
Amplitude	> 5 mm and <25 mm in limb leads; 5 to 30 mm in V_1 and V_6; 7 to 30 mm in V_2 and V_5; 9 to 30 mm in V_3 and V_4
R progression	Progressive rise in R wave amplitude from V_1 to V_6
Axis	−30 to + 120 degrees
Transition	V_3 or V_4

Component	Criteria
Intrinsicoid deflection	<0.02 sec in V_1; <0.04 sec in V_6 Delayed in BBB and chamber enlargement

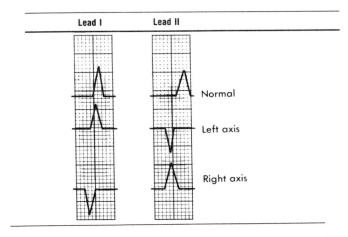

Component	Criteria
U wave	
Direction	Upright
Amplitude	0.33 mm in precordial leads (average); 2.5 mm (maximum) Increases in amplitude in hypokalemia
Width	<0.24 sec

D. *Recognizing Axis*

	Lead I	Lead II	
			Normal
			Left axis
			Right axis

E. Differentiating BBB

LBBB	RBBB
V_1: $-$QRS complex	V_1: rSR′
V_6: $+$QRS complex	V_1: Intrinsicoid deflection 0.07 sec or later in V_1
I, aVL, V_6: R wave, no Q wave, no S wave	I, aVL, V_6: broad S wave, small Q

F. Differentiating Hemiblock

Anterior hemiblock	Posterior hemiblock
LAD >-40	RAD $+120$
QRS duration: normal	II, III, aVF: Q waves
I, aVL: small Q waves	I, aVL: R wave
II, III: small initial R waves	

G. Quick Guide to Evaluate Broad QRS Tachycardia

Look at lead V_1, if QRS pattern is mainly positive, the following characteristics favor VT:

Monophasic or biphasic QRS

R to S ratio <1 (deep S wave) in V_6

Left rabbit ear taller in V_1

Look at lead V_1-V_2; if QRS pattern is mainly negative, the following characteristics favor VT (Figure 18):

Broad R (>0.03 sec)

Slurred/notched downslope of S

>0.06 sec from R to nadir of S wave

any Q in V_6

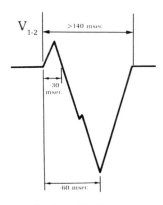

Fig. 18 Broad QRS pattern in V_1-V_2.

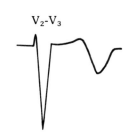

Fig. 19 ECG findings with critical stenosis of proximal LAD.

H. *Wellen's Syndrome*

Signs associated with critical stenosis of proximal LAD and impending infarction:

History: positive for prior angina

Laboratory: little or no cardiac enzyme elevation

ECG: no pathological precordial Q wave

V_2-V_3: ST segment turns down into a negative T at an angle of 60-90 degrees; deeply inverted symmetrical T wave (Figure 19)

I. *Types of Infarctions*

Type of infarction	Anatomical location	ECG patterns
Lateral		I, aV$_L$, V$_5$, V$_6$: abnormal Q wave, ST elevation, T wave inversion
Inferior		II, III, aV$_F$: abnormal Q wave, ST elevation, T wave inversion
Anterior		V$_1$-V$_4$; abnormal Q wave, loss of R wave progression, ST elevation, T wave inversion
Posterior		V$_1$, V$_2$: tall R wave, ST depression, tall symmetrical T wave
NOTE: RV infarction		V$_4$R: ST elevation >1 mm

SECTION IV PEDIATRIC ASSESSMENT GUIDES

I. PEDIATRIC VITAL SIGNS

	6 mo	1 yr	3 yr	6 yr	10 yr
Heart rate (beats/min)	90-120	90-120	80-120	70-110	60-90
Respirations (breaths/min)	25-40	20-30	20-30	18-25	15-20
Systolic blood pressure (mm Hg)	80-100	80-100	80-110	80-110	90-120

II. PEDIATRIC COMA SCALE

Eye opening:	Spontaneous	4
	To speech	3
	To pain	2
	No response	1
Best motor response:	Spontaneous	6
	Localizes pain	5
	Withdraws to pain	4
	Flexes to pain	3
	Extends to pain	2
	No response	1
Best verbal response: (use if 4 yr of age or older)	Oriented	5
	Confused	4
	Inappropriate	3
	Incomprehensible	2
	No response	1
Best response to auditory/ visual stimulus: (use if 3 yr of age or younger)	Smiles, oriented to sound, follows objects, interacts	5
	Crying is consolable, interacts inappropriately	4
	Moans, is inconsistently con- solable, is irritable	3
	Is inconsolable, restless	2
	No response	1

III RECOGNIZING SIGNS AND SYMPTOMS OF DISTRESS

A. *Manifestations of Increased Intracranial Pressure*
- Change in level of consciousness
- Dilated pupils with sluggish reaction to light
- Abnormal motor activity
- Abnormal reflexes

B. *Manifestations of Respiratory Distress in the Child*
- Tachypnea, bradypnea is an ominous sign
- Increased respiratory effort (retractions, nasal flaring, head bobbing with each breath, seesaw respirations)
- Diminished breath sounds, stridor, wheezing, grunting
- Decreased level of consciousness
- Decreased/poor skeletal muscle tone
- Cyanosis (late sign)

C. *Signs Indicative of Cardiovascular Decompensation and Decreased End-Organ Perfusion*
- Tachycardia
- Bradycardia (impending cardiac arrest)
- Drop in systolic blood pressure (10 mm Hg) accompanied by an increased heart rate (late sign of shock)
- Descrepancy in volume between central and peripheral pulses
- Narrowed pulse pressure (systolic minus diastolic blood pressure)
- Decreased skin perfusion (skin temperature, color)
- Prolonged capillary refill
- Decreased central nervous system perfusion (altered level of consciousness; decreasing response to verbal stimuli, pain; depressed deep tendon reflexes; change in pupil size)
- Decreased urine output (<1-2 ml/kg/hr)

IV. MISCELLANEOUS FORMULAS

A. *Estimation of Systolic Blood Pressure (SBP) and Diastolic Blood Pressure (DBP)*

SBP = 2 × age + 80

DBP = ⅔ of SBP

B. *Estimation of Patient Weight in Kilograms*

kg = 8 + (age × 2)

C. *Estimation of Endotracheal (ET) Tube Size*

$$ET \text{ size} = \frac{16 + age}{4}$$

D. *Estimation of Fluid Bolus*

10-20 ml/kg

V. DAILY FLUID MAINTENANCE REQUIREMENTS

Weight	Requirement
0-10 kg	100 ml/kg
11-20 kg	1000 ml/day *plus*
	50 ml/kg for each kg 11 through 20
21-30 kg	1500 ml/day *plus*
	25 ml/kg for each kg 21 through 30
31-40 kg	1750 ml/day *plus*
	10 ml/kg for each kg 31 through 40

VI. PEDIATRIC SIZES FOR RESUSCITATION EQUIPMENT

Age	Wt (kg)	Laryngoscope	ETT (mm)	Suction (Fr)	CT (Fr)	NG (Fr)	Foley (Fr)
0-6 mo	3-5	0	3.0	6	10-12	8	5
6-12 mo	7	1	3.5	6	10-12	8	5
1 yr	10	1	3.5	8	16-20	8	8
18 mo	12	1	4.0	8	16-20	8	8
3 yr	15	2	4.5	10	16-20	10	10
5 yr	20	2	5.0	10	20-28	10	10
6 yr	20	2	5.5	10	20-28	10	10
8 yr	25	2	6.0	10	20-28	10	10
10 yr	30	2	6.0	10	28-32	12	12
12 yr	40	2	6.5	14	28-32	12	12
14 yr	50	3	7.0	14	32-42	14	12

ETT, Endotracheal tube; *CT*, chest tube
NG, nasogastric.

VII. EMERGENCY PEDIATRIC PHARMACOLOGY
A. Emergency Drug Dosages

Drug	Usual IV dose
Atropine	0.02 mg/kg
Bretylium	Initial: 5 mg/kg
	Repeat: 10 mg/kg
Calcium chloride 10%	20 mg/kg (0.2 ml/kg)
Dextrose 50%	500 mg/kg
Diazepam	0.1 mg/kg
Epinephrine	0.01 mg/kg of 1:10,000 solution
Ketamine	1-2 mg/kg (normovolemia)
	0.5 mg/kg (hypovolemia)
Lidocaine	1 mg/kg
Naloxone	0.01 mg/kg
Phenobarbital	20 mg/kg
Phenytoin	15 mg/kg
Procainamide	5 mg/kg
Propranolol	0.1 mg/kg
Sodium bicarbonate	1 mEq/kg
Verapamil	0.1 mg/kg

B. *Continuous Infusions*

Drug	Range (μg/kg/min)
Alprostadil	0.1-0.4
Dobutamine	2-20
Dopamine	2-20
Epinephrine	0.1-1.0
Isoproterenol	0.1-1.0
Lidocaine	20-50
Nitroglycerin	1-25
Nitroprusside	1-8
Norepinephrine	0.1-1.0

SECTION V LABORATORY VALUES

I. BLOOD STUDIES
A. *Complete Blood Count*

RBC	$4.25\text{-}5.5 \times 10^6/\mu l$ (males)
	$3.6\text{-}5.0 \times 10^6/\mu l$ (females)
WBC	$5\text{-}10 \times 10^3/\mu l$
Hgb	13.5-17.5 g/dl (males)
	12-16 g/dl (females)
Hct	40%-54% (males)
	37%-47% (females)

B. *Coagulation*

Platelets	$150\text{-}350 \times 10^3/\mu l$
PT	10-14 sec
PTT	30-45 sec
APTT	16-25 sec
ACT	92-128 sec
FSP	$<10 \ \mu g/dl$

C. *Chemistry*

Na	135-148 mEq/L
K	3.5-5.0 mEq/L
Cl	98-106 mEq/L
CO_2	24-32 mEq/L

BUN	7-18 mg/dl
Cr	0.7-1.3 mg/dl (males)
	0.6-1.2 mg/dl (females)
Glucose	70-110 mg/dl
Ca	8.5-10.5 mg/dl
Mg	1.3-2.1 mEq/L
Osmolality	275-295 mOsm/kg
Bilirubin	
Direct	0-0.2 mg/dl
Total	0.2-1.0 mg/dl
Indirect	total minus direct
Amylase	50-150 U/L
Lipase	4-24 U/L
Anion gap	8-16 mEq/L
Lactate	0.5-2.2 mEq/L

D. Cardiac Profile

SGOT (AST)	6-18 U/L (females)
	7-21 U/L (males)
With MI	
Onset:	12-18 hours
Peak:	24-48 hours
Duration:	3-4 days
CK	96-140 U/L (females)
	38-174 U/L (males)
With MI	
Onset:	4-6 hours
Peak:	12-24 hours
Duration:	3-4 days

CK-MB	0%
With MI	
Onset:	4-6 hours
Peak:	12-24 hours
Duration:	2-3 days
LDH	90-200 U/L
With MI	
Onset:	24-48 hours
Peak:	3-6 days
Duration:	7-10 days
LDH_1	17.5-28.3% of total LDH
LDH_2	30.4-36.4% of total LDH
With MI	
$LDH_1 > LDH_2$	
Onset:	12-24 hours
Peak:	48 hours
Duration:	variable

II. MISCELLANEOUS
A. Urine Electrolytes

Na	40-220 mEq/L
K	25-125 mEq/L
Cl	110-250 mEq/L

B. *Drug Levels*

Digoxin	1-2 ng/ml
Phenytoin	10-20 µg/ml
Theophylline	10-20 µg/ml
Barbiturate coma	10 mg/100 ml
Gentamicin	
Trough	1-2 µg/ml
Peak	6-8 µg/ml
Tobramycin	
Trough	1-2 µg/ml
Peak	6-8 µg/ml

SECTION VI FORMULAS AND CONVERSION FACTORS

MISCELLANEOUS CALCULATIONS

$\mu g/ml = mg/ml \times 1000$

$ml/min = ml/hr \div 60$

$\mu g/kg/min = \dfrac{\mu g/ml \times ml/min}{wt(kg)}$

$ml/hr = \dfrac{wt(kg) \times \mu g/kg/min}{\mu g/ml} \times 60$

CONVERSION FACTORS

1 kg	= 1 liter fluid	1/150 gr	= 0.4 mg
1 mg	= 1000 μg	1 tsp	= 5 ml
1 kg	= 2.2 lb	1 Tbsp	= 15 ml
1 gr	= 60 mg	1 oz	= 30 ml
1/100 gr	= 0.6 mg	1 mm Hg	= 1.36 cm H_2O

Parameter	Formula	Normal range
Alveolar-arterial oxygen gradient ($AaDO_2$)	$PAo_2 - Pao_2$	< 15 mm Hg
Alveolar partial pressure of oxygen (PAo_2)	$FiO_2 (713) - PaCO_2/0.8$	
Anion gap (GAP)	$Na - (HCO_3 + Cl)$	8-16 mEq/L
Arterial oxygen content (CaO_2)	$(SaO_2 \times Hgb \times 1.34) + (PaO_2 \times .0031)$	18-20 ml/100 ml or 20 vol %
Arterial oxygen delivery (DO_2)	$CO \times 10 \times CaO_2$	900-1200 ml/min
Arterial venous oxygen content difference ($C_{(a-v)}O_2$)	$CaO_2 - CvO_2$	4-6 ml/100 ml or vol %
Cardiac index (CI)	$\dfrac{CO}{BSA}$	2.5-4.0 L/min/m^2
Cardiac output (CO)	$HR \times SV$	4-8 L/min
Cerebral perfusion pressure (CPP)	$MAP - ICP$	80-100 mm Hg

Continued.

Parameter	Formula	Normal range
Coronary perfusion pressure (CPP)	DBP − PAWP	60-80 mm Hg
Ejection fraction (EF)	$\dfrac{SV}{\text{end diastolic volume}} \times 100$	60% or greater
Glomerular filtration rate (GRF)	$\dfrac{(140 - \text{Age}) \times \text{wt(kg)}}{\text{(male) } 75 \times \text{serum Cr}}$ (female) $85 \times$ serum Cr	80-120 ml/min
Intracranial pressure (ICP)		0-15 mm Hg
Left ventricular stroke work index (LVSWI)	(MAP − PAWP)SVI × 0.136	45-60 g-m/m^2
Mean arterial pressure (MAP)	$\dfrac{2(DBP) + SBP}{3}$	70-105 mm Hg
Osmolality (OSM)	(2Na) + K + BUN/3 + Glucose/18	275-295 mOsm
Oxygen consumption (VO$_2$)	CO × 10 × C$_{(a-v)}$O$_2$	200-250 ml/min
Pulmonary vascular resistance (PVR)	$\dfrac{\text{PAM} - \text{PAWP}}{\text{CO}} \times 80$	100-250 dynes/sec/cm^{-5}

Parameter	Formula	Normal value
Pulmonary vascular resistance index (PVRI)	$\dfrac{\text{PAM} - \text{PAWP}}{\text{CI}} \times 80$	200-450 dynes/sec/cm^{-5}/m^2
Rate pressure product (RPP)	HR $\times$ SBP	<12,000
Respiratory quotient (RQ)	$\dfrac{CO_2 \text{ production}}{O_2 \text{ consumption}}$	0.8-1
Right ventricular stroke work index (RVSWI)	(PAM $-$ CVP)SVI $\times$ 0.136	8.5-12 g-m/m^2
Stroke volume (SV)	$\dfrac{\text{CO} \times 1000}{\text{HR}}$	60-80 ml/beat
Stroke volume index (SVI)	$\dfrac{\text{SV}}{\text{BSA}}$ or $\dfrac{\text{CI}}{\text{HR}} \times 1000$	40-50 ml/m^2/beat
Systemic vascular resistance (SVR)	$\dfrac{\text{MAP} - \text{CVP}}{\text{CO}} \times 80$	900-1400 dynes/sec/cm^{-5}
Systemic vascular resistance index (SVRI)	$\dfrac{\text{MAP} - \text{CVP}}{\text{CI}} \times 80$	1700-2600 dynes/sec/cm^{-5}/m^2
Venous oxygen content (CvO$_2$)	(SvO$_2$ $\times$ Hgb $\times$ 1.34) + (PvO$_2$ $\times$ .0031)	15.5 ml/100 ml or vol %

FIGURES AND TABLES ARE REPRINTED WITH PERMISSION FROM THE FOLLOWING SOURCES:

Budassi SA: *Mosby's manual of emergency care,* ed 3, St Louis, 1990, Mosby.

Conover M: *Pocket guide to electrocardiography,* ed 2, St Louis, 1990, Mosby.

Conover M: *Understanding electrocardiography,* ed 6, St Louis, 1992, Mosby.

Daily E, Schroeder J: *Hemodynamic waveforms,* ed 2, St Louis, 1990, Mosby.

Kinney M et al: *Comprehensive cardiac care,* ed 7, St Louis, 1991, Mosby.

Kinney M et al: *AACN's clinical reference for critical care nursing,* ed 3, St Louis, 1993, Mosby.

Seidel H: *Mosby's guide to physical examination,* ed 2, St Louis, 1991, Mosby.

Stillwell S: *Mosby's critical care nursing reference,* St Louis, 1992, Mosby.

Stillwell S, Randall E: *Pocket guide to cardiovascular care,* St Louis, 1990, Mosby.

Talbot L, Marquardt M: *Pocket guide to critical care assessment,* St Louis, 1993, Mosby.

Thelan L et al: *Textbook of critical care nursing,* ed 2, St Louis, 1993, Mosby.